Basic Yoga Guide

Different Styles of Yoga for All Ages

Jesse Simonds

Copyright © [2023] by [JESSE SIMONDS]

TABLE OF CONTENTS

INTRODUCTION

Firstly, I would like to say how appreciative I am that you picked up this book. Physically, yoga consists of a series of poses or stretches that have their origins in Indian and Hindu philosophy, but it is also much more than that. These "asanas" (the English version) or "poses" (the original Sanskrit term) can improve your physical health, mental clarity, and emotional equilibrium. They are commonly known to improve circulation, which in turn aids in eliminating waste products, honing mental faculties, and releasing emotional blocks. There's evidence that they do the same for the soul as well. While the exact beginnings of yoga cannot be pinpointed, scholars estimate that it has been practiced for at least five thousand years.

Modern yoga is a relatively new iteration of an old discipline. Modern yoga, which originated in India and made its way to the United States in the early 20th century, is a synthesis of old Indian cultural practices and asanas with gymnastics, physical therapy, and naturopathy. The goal of modern yoga is to assist its practitioners get more in touch with themselves, their bodies, and their emotions and intuitions. At the same time, you get a complete body exercise with both strength training and stretching. Although some people have incorporated yoga into their religious rituals, yoga is not a religion in and of itself. That's hardly surprising, given that this type of physical activity is excellent for reducing stress, easing anxiety, and facilitating mental clarity—all of which are necessary for developing one's spirituality. However, the mental and emotional benefits of physical yoga practice are the primary focus of this book.

The bulk of yoga postures are glandular system stimulators, meaning they help your internal organs work better. The deep, controlled breathing practiced during this form of exercise contributes to the development of a tranquil, attentive state of mind. Consistent yoga practice has been linked to numerous positive effects on a person's body, mind, and spirit.

While we will go into greater detail about the potential benefits of yoga in the following chapter, here are some of the things you can expect to gain from practicing the poses presented in this book. Yoga:

1 Prevents a wide variety of health problems, from headaches to cardiovascular disease.

2 Builds and maintains a sturdy skeleton.

3 Improves one's state of mind and facilitates the operation of the nervous system and other "invisible" bodyparts.

4 Is a cheap method of boosting your emotional, physical, and spiritual wellness.

5 Can be picked up quickly and easily.

6 Can be done by almost anyone, in any setting.

There is a wide spectrum of yoga practices and levels of complexity, from the easiest to the most challenging. You've definitely heard of Yoga, but your knowledge likely stops with Hatha Yoga, the most common kind. Posture, motion, and breathing are the main areas of concentration. Some forms of yoga place a heavy emphasis on meditative breathing and reflective thought, while others highlight religious wisdom and tradition. However, the mental and physical benefits of Hatha Yoga are what this book will center on.

It's Yoga Time!

Adults of any age or fitness level can benefit from practicing yoga. As you'll see, this book is filled with warnings about which postures you should avoid if you have a preexisting medical problem. Changes can be made to practice other positions. If a certain yoga pose makes you feel uneasy, pay attention to that sensation and investigate why you might be experiencing it.

The connections between your thoughts, feelings, and physical self are all interdependent. Both will be impacted by the events that occur. When one's feelings are unresponsive to therapy, it is not unusual for that person to seek medical help. The same holds true for bodily ailments: if yoga isn't helping, it might be time to see a doctor.

If you are concerned that your yoga postures could be causing you harm or preventing you from reaping the full benefits of a particular pose, it may be worthwhile to consult a certified yoga instructor. However, if you adhere to the instructions and respect the limitations that are given for each pose, practicing the beginner-level poses in this book is unlikely to cause any harm. You are welcome to use these pages as a jumping off point into the rewarding and taxing practice of yoga.

Girls and Ladies

Most yoga instructors agree that inversions and other challenging positions should be avoided by pregnant and nursing women, but they also acknowledge that softer asanas, such as child's pose, can be beneficial. A woman's body goes through a lot during her reproductive years, and this book has poses that can help with everything from monthly cramps to menopause symptoms to providing comfort during pregnancy.

To prevent back pain and injuries from the strain of raising and carrying a baby, nursing women can benefit from poses that offer support to the muscles needed to hold a baby when breastfeeding. In addition to helping mom and baby relax during those first few weeks of breastfeeding, it can also assist mom deal with postpartum depression. Some moms even choose to feed their babies while doing yoga.

Prenatal yoga is a great approach for expectant mothers to maintain their fitness levels. Your yoga teacher will be able to modify your routine as your pregnancy develops, and they can advise you on which asanas to practice to prepare your body for labor and delivery.

A consultation with a certified yoga teacher is advised in each of these scenarios. With the help of an expert, you can improve the quality and safety of your yoga practice through modifications to existing poses and the introduction of new ones.

Yoga may be a lot of fun for kids of all ages to play around with their friends and family members. A child's self-awareness and self-control can both benefit from the breathing exercises. Only the same risks as those faced by young gymnasts exist. Instead of helping children's developing bodies, excessive exercise that goes beyond what is pleasurable and natural can actually do more harm than good. However, most kids find yoga to be a delightful way to play.

How to Begin

Yoga can be studied in numerous different ways. Learning from a qualified instructor in the company of other students is a popular choice. You can learn yoga via a video if you don't have the time or money to attend a class. To further your yoga practice, you can even play an interactive video game.

The third alternative is to educate oneself. You can easily train yourself using the text and visual aids included in this book, while periodic consultation with an experienced instructor is recommended.

Here you can find tried-and-true, step-by-step instructions for the most common and widely beneficial yoga postures. To help you reap yoga's many rewards, these directions cover breathing exercises and mental preparation. There is no missing information; you may jump right into the basics.

You will gain an understanding of how to prepare your body for yoga and will rapidly become proficient in the foundational mountain position. All of the yoga postures can be mastered with the help of the detailed instructions provided throughout this book. You'll also learn a wide range of positions that target certain areas of your body.

In addition, you'll get guidance on creating a sustainable home practice of yoga, from the fundamentals to more advanced techniques. At the end of the book, I provide five different yoga routines that each target a different set of issues. After this, there's a whole chapter devoted to tailoring your yoga routine to your own physical, mental, emotional, and even spiritual demands. Also included are suggestions for incorporating yoga into your daily routine. You'll find that yoga has a wide range of positive effects.

Yoga is a wonderful practice to try because it can be done anywhere, costs next to nothing, and offers only benefits. You can get started with just a comfortable outfit. Even a yoga mat is optional; it serves only to provide a clean surface with some padding and to keep your body from slipping out of position.

If you find that yoga is something you really like doing, you might want to get some new gear down the road. Using a blanket as a prop can help you achieve deeper stretches and hold poses for longer. Yoga straps and blocks are used to assist with connecting the hands or bridging the gap between the hands and feet in various positions. Don't allow the lack of these things stop you, though; as I stated, they're not necessary. Let's go in right now.

CHAPTER 1

TIPS FOR DESIGNING YOUR OWN YOGA ROUTINE

Methods of Yoga Sequencing

You may have reached the point where you feel comfortable with the sequence I've created for you, but you may not be ready to enroll in a studio lesson just yet.

Don't worry; I'll protect you. In this chapter, we'll discuss the steps necessary to design and implement a customized yoga workout routine.

Here's the Way to Get It Done

It's both exciting and nerve-wracking to create your own yoga regimen for the first time. The ability to tailor a workout to specific needs and objectives is unparalleled.

Many yoga students prefer to take lessons because they have no idea how to practice the discipline on their own. Well, I'm here to tell you that you don't need an instructor to benefit from yoga, and that you can create your own routine right now.

Now we begin...

Step 1: Grab a scrap of paper and a pen, because you're going to want to make a list of all your favorite yoga poses. Identifying yoga poses in a way that makes sense to you is more important than knowing the correct name or Sanskrit term for each position. Your selection could be brief or extensive. If it's too brief and you're hoping to build a more extensive practice, you could want to look into yoga books and publications for inspiration on more positions.

Step 2: Group similar poses together, then further categorize them by whether they are inversions, twists, arm balances, forward bends, standing, restoratives, or backbends. You could go quite specific about which muscles are being worked (legs, arms, core, etc.) if you wanted to.

You should do poses from each category to create a well-rounded routine. Before you start your workout, write down the number of Sun Salutations you intend to do.

Step 3: Remember that the Basic Breath Awareness technique should come first in your workout (even before the Sun Salutations). It's so crucial that you should always do this. However, with time and effort, you should be able to slow your breathing down much more quickly. Find a peaceful place where you can sit still and concentrate on your breathing for at least five minutes.

Step 4: Developing your own exercise program is to determine whether you want to emphasize restorative, restorative and strengthening, or restorative and energizing exercises.

It's crucial that the positions you choose reflect your desired aesthetic. For instance, if your goal is to unwind, you should focus on seated or lying-down poses like the Child's

Pose. Inversions, arm balances, and even backbends are all great ways to improve strength.

Finally, if you want to feel revitalized, focus on a more dynamic sequence like the Sun Salutations or the Warrior Poses, Half Moon Pose, Triangle Pose, etc.

Step 5: In my opinion, the most crucial part of the whole process. Unfortunately, when we get to this part of our yoga routine, I often see students running away from their mats, which is a shame because it is so important to our well-being.

Please explain. Savasana, also known as the Corpse Pose, is a resting posture that should be practiced at the end of every single one of your yoga sessions. Even if it isn't a part of the routine!

In order to properly digest and reflect on the journey we've just completed, it's important to give your body and mind some time to rest and recuperate after the intense activities of the last hour or so.

The five minutes you spend lying on your mat at the end of your workout, breathing deeply and relaxing thoroughly, will be well worth it.

That settles it, then! These 5 components are necessary for creating a personalized yoga routine.

And if you find your groove, you might even want to become a Certified Yoga Teacher and help others do the same!

CHAPTER 2

THERAPEUTIC YOGA

Overworked muscles, joints, ligaments, and tendons require rest and repair after any kind of athletic or physical exercise. Yoga may not be as "physically demanding" as other sports like football.

When you don't give your body the time it needs to recover from the stress of repeated motion, you run the risk of injuring the same muscles and joints in new ways.

However, with yoga, you won't need to take a day off; in fact, there are yoga practices that are designed specifically to relieve the soreness and stiffness that can result from overuse. Stress can come from anywhere: a strenuous profession, an extreme activity, or even other forms of yoga (such Vinyasa Flow or Power Yoga).

Healing Yoga Positions

I highly recommend taking a class the first few times you try restorative yoga, if you find yourself in need of some relaxation. Why? We don't need any more injuries, and you'll get more out of the practice if you master the poses the right way the first time.

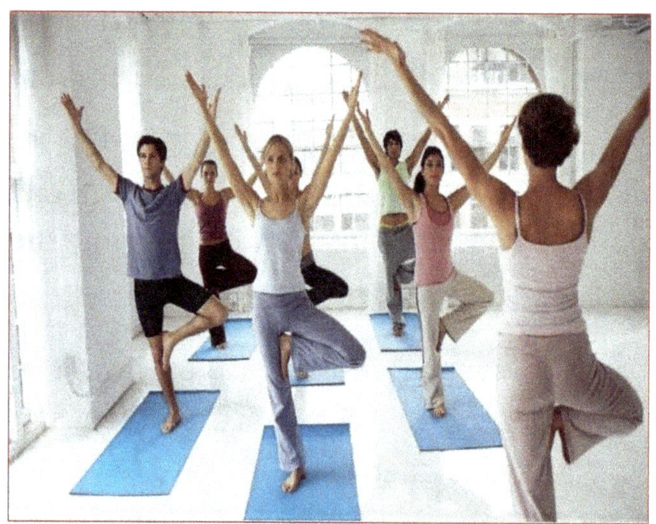

The fact that restorative yoga is akin to taking a nap is one of its many appealing features. Your instructor will lead you through a series of restorative postures designed to relieve the mental strain caused by the mundane tasks we must all perform. When someone else is "thinking" for you and guiding your ideas in the appropriate direction, you can get a lot more done.

It's highly unlikely that anyone who tries restorative yoga for the first time in a group session will ever want to do it any other way.

CHAPTER 3

THE FOUNDATIONS OF ORIENTAL YOGA

The saying goes, "Nature wastes no time, yet manages to get everything done."

— Lao Tzu

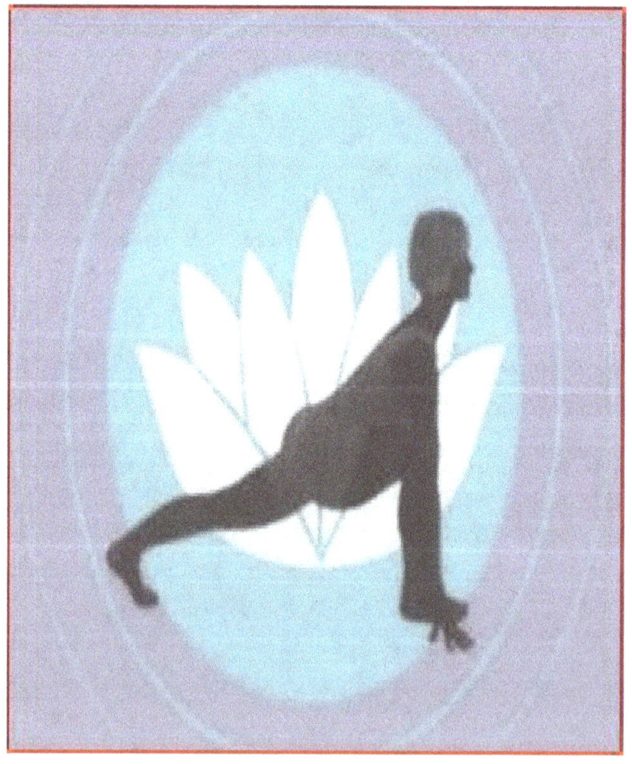

An Overview of the Five Phases and Elements

The 5 element theory of Traditional Chinese Medicine and Taoist cosmology was probably developed between 476 and 221 BC. One of the earliest steps toward what we now call science was taken when people realized that natural phenomena did not originate from supernatural beings who wreaked havoc on Earth when they were angry or showered gifts from on high when they were pleased, but rather were the result of the interplay between various natural elements.

This changed their entire perspective on life and the causes of illness. They gradually honed in on five fundamental ingredients and the interconnections among all physical events, based largely on their own observations. They also made linkages between these factors and the human mind, heart, and soul. This viewpoint did not go away with the passing of time. Instead, it got even more entrenched in the theory and practice of traditional Chinese medicine and Taoism, making it one of the world's oldest and most tried-and-true medical systems.

Let's examine these five parts more thoroughly:

They are the 5 Elements:

1 Stomach and Spleen - Earth, Late Summer
2 Alloy - fall - The Lungs and the Big Stomach
3 Liquid - Cold - Kidneys and Bladder
4 Hearth, spring, the Liver, and Gallbladder are all made of Wood.
5 Heart, ileum, pericardium, and San Jiao (thermostat) are under the purview of the Fire element during the summerseason.

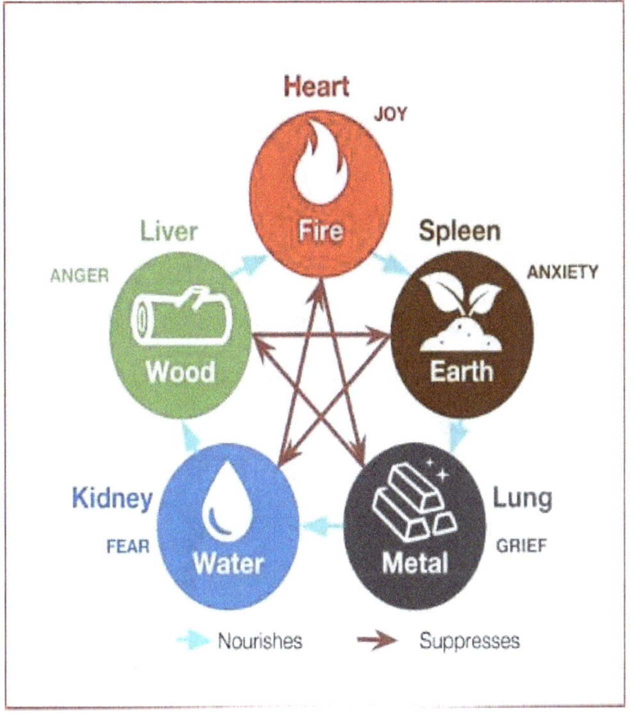

There are two distinct relationships at play. The Shen cycle is concerned with nurturing, while the Ko cycle is concerned with exerting control.

The Shen Cycle (The Art of Caring) Exposed

The Shen is characterized as the cycle of generation and nurturing, like that between a mother and her son. There is a circular movement of energy from one part to another. The next element is negatively impacted when energy becomes locked, stagnant, or weak in the previous element. The Earth element can be negatively affected if, for instance, the Fire element becomes obstructed or sluggish, or if the fire itself is extinguished or smothered. Then, the Earth element will start showing symptoms of illness, and restoring the Shen cycle will necessitate treating the Fire element in tandem with the Earth element.

The Ko Cycle (of Control) Exposed

The relationship between a grandmother and a grandson, at least in conventional households, is seen as analogous to the Ko cycle, which is why it is sometimes called the controlling cycle. The grandson's grandmother is a major figure in his life. Applying the same logic as in the Shen case, where the Earth element had become weak and there were symptoms associated with this, we might conclude that the Wood element was responsible for Earth's problems. Because the liver is so easily irritated by heat, the Wood element can easily dominate the Earth. Or, the Wood element could be deliberately withholding energy from the Earth element, leaving the Earth in a precarious position. Therefore, there are times when Wood element treatment is required in order to effect change in Earth element treatment, and so on.

Although it is not essential to fully understand these concepts, doing so will be very helpful when treating any illness or signs of imbalance. Understanding the connections between the parts helps us zero in on the likely origin of the issue, which is crucial for getting to the root of the problem rather than just treating the symptoms.

It's all about Yin and Yang and the Whole Shi-bang!

The yin and yang? Which part does this play? According to traditional Chinese philosophy, yin and yang are the initial manifestations of energy from the all-pervasive ONE, or Wuji. Qi (a highly intelligent, electrical fabric, also frequently referred to as bioenergy) was the form of energy that emanated from the primal ONE. To manifest, it had to cut off its connection to the UNITED STATES, resulting in the polar opposites of yin and yang. We Westerners have given it the names yin and yang, and it may look like a split power to us, but this is only partially accurate. It is an expression of the UNITED source, not a division of it. Separating it into yin and yang allows humans to more easily discuss and understand it. The universe of yin and yang is a world of opposites: of day and night, of the sun and the moon, of good and evil, of words and divisions, of ideas and concepts. This Qi power, which initially manifested as yin and yang, then separated into the five elements to form the material universe. Despite the fact that their physical bodies are composed of the five elements, their minds are dominated by thought, which is inherently dualistic in nature (yin and yang), and their hearts are linked to the ONE or the Wuji, many humans remain oblivious to these facts.

Humanity's over-focus on logic and the yin and yang of things is a major roadblock on the path to enlightenment. To some extent, it is helpful to tap into and comprehend the yin and yang of our world and our minds.

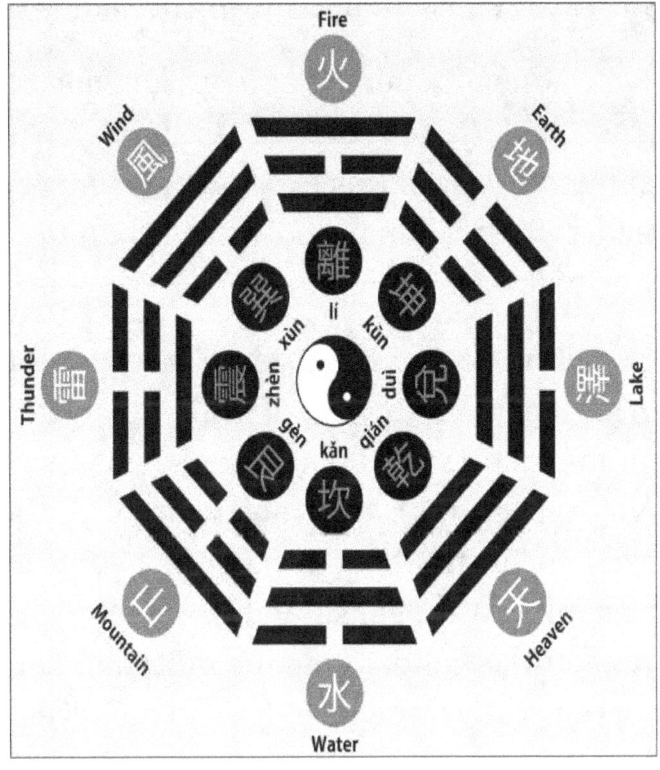

Nonetheless, man lacks the belief and experience necessary to cultivate and nurture the relationship with the source that resides in the heart, and this disconnection lessens one's capacity to live fully. All those who have attained enlightenment have established themselves firmly in the source, the field beyond yin and yang, beyond the confines of the mind. While one's physical form will perpetually be subject to the 5 elements, one's spiritual self is not necessarily bound by them.

When a person's physical, mental, and emotional states are in harmony with the universal flow of this expression of energy, he is said to be walking the Tao, or the Way of the spiritual warrior.

The goal of the Oriental Yoga system is to bring harmony to the 5 elements, cleanse the mind, and expand emotional capacity. Asana (yogic postures), diet, and way of life are all used to bring about a balance between the 5 elements. We cleanse and balance the yin and yang of the mind through meditation and other contemplative practices. The true ONE of the cosmos can enter through the door of the heart once the mental and material worlds have been cleansed and brought into harmony. The method entails constant cleansing and cultivation of mind and matter harmony to enlarge this gateway and solidify the passage to the heart. The influence of the 5 elements and the intellectualizing mind will gradually fade as one becomes firmly rooted on the path of the heart. But first, try to calm and cleanse your mind by working to bring balance to the five elements. The rest will become clear to the practitioner at the appropriate time.

Auras, Chakras, and Meridians

Entering the realm of "energetic anatomy," we learn about the Chakras and the meridians. In traditional Indian yogic traditions, the Chakras are described as large energy centers, wheels, or vortices where massive amounts of Qi energy are processed and generated. Human beings have seven major chakras, or energy centers, spread out along their spinal column. According to Yoga, the meridian channels, also known as "Nadi" channels, are responsible for transporting Qi from the Chakras to the rest of the body. Because of this mutual dependence, it is essential to take into account both the Chakras and the meridian channels simultaneously throughout any therapeutic procedure.

Although most people can't see the Chakras with their naked eyes, they can usually sense and feel them unconsciously and consciously. The Chakras are extremely potent and can affect not only the physical but also the mental, emotional, and spiritual aspects of a person.

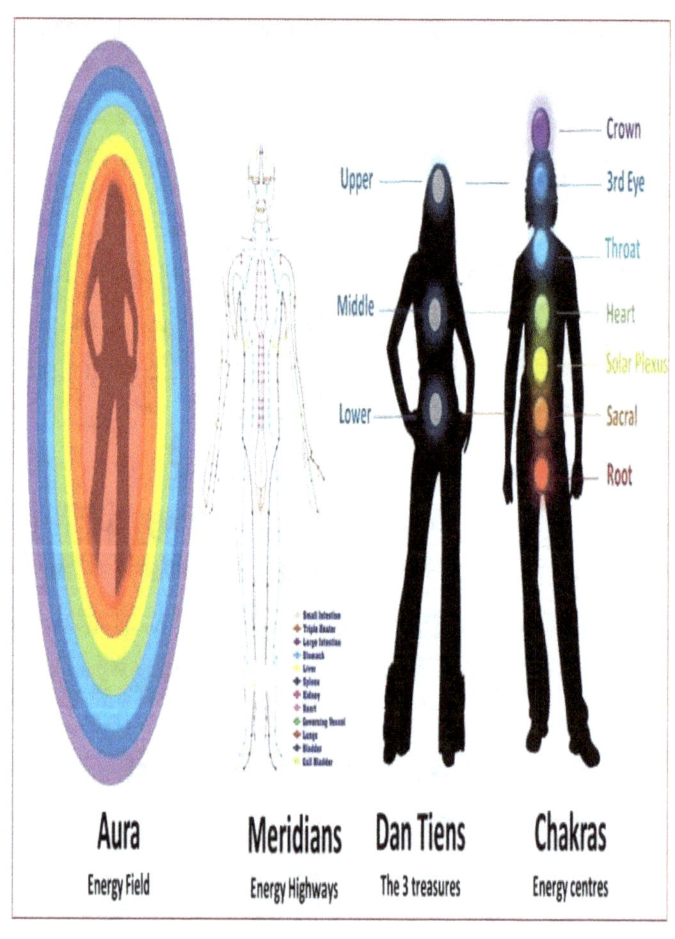

The meridians are an extensive system of energy channels responsible for transporting Qi and blood throughout the body.

Like a river system, they carry vital nutrients throughout the body and energy system, ensuring that everything is always working at peak efficiency. Any disruption to the meridian or Chakra systems can lead to a wide variety of symptoms on the physical, mental, and spiritual planes. Taoists from ancient China zeroed in on the 14 primary channel pathways still used in modern TCM, meticulously charting each one. Both this book and the vast majority of other works on Oriental medicine depict meridian pathways primarily at the points at which they exit the body. These meridians extend their networks deep within the body, which is important to keep in mind. Because of their convenient proximity to the skin's surface, we tend to prioritize treating conditions that manifest in these channels.

Herbal medicines, herbal tinctures, diet, and meditative practices are recommended because they have better access to the internal environment and can therefore treat the deeper networks of these meridians, which is especially important when dealing with certain illnesses that are said to be very internalized.

The meridians of each organ serve to nourish, feed, and express that organ specifically. Three of these meridians don't serve any particular organ but are important for energy flow nonetheless. The lungs, the large intestine, the kidneys, the bladder, the liver, the gallbladder, the heart, the pericardium, the small intestine, the stomach, and the spleen are all connected to meridians. The central Ren, the back Du, and the temperature regulator San Jiao are the three extra meridians.

The primary focus of Oriental Yoga is on the 14 major meridians, with some attention also paid to the 3 primary chakras. The second Chakra (called Hara in Japan and dan tien in China), the fourth Chakra (called Shen in Chinese medicine), and the sixth Chakra (called the third eye in Western medicine) are the three main energy centers in the body.

An Overview of the Oriental Dietary Approach

Food is treated very differently in Oriental diet treatment than it is in the West. One of the guiding concepts, particularly if eating only well-cooked foods such soups, stews, casseroles, and porridges, and drinking only warm tea and warm water, is recommended for those who are sick or weak. Foods that have already been cooked and are easily digested are best because they provide the body with the nutrients it needs without needing it to use too much energy. It is widely held that different foods and plants have different warming and cooling characteristics, and that they must be taken into account when planning a diet to achieve optimal health. In relation to the seasons, we can get away with eating cooler foods like salads, fruits, and raw foods in the summer and spring when there is a lot of heat in the atmosphere and it is also transferred into our bodies. The body needs more cooked, warm foods in the winter and fall to keep it nourished and warm. Ice cold beverages, water, and foods like ice cream should be avoided, especially in colder areas or when feeling under the weather.

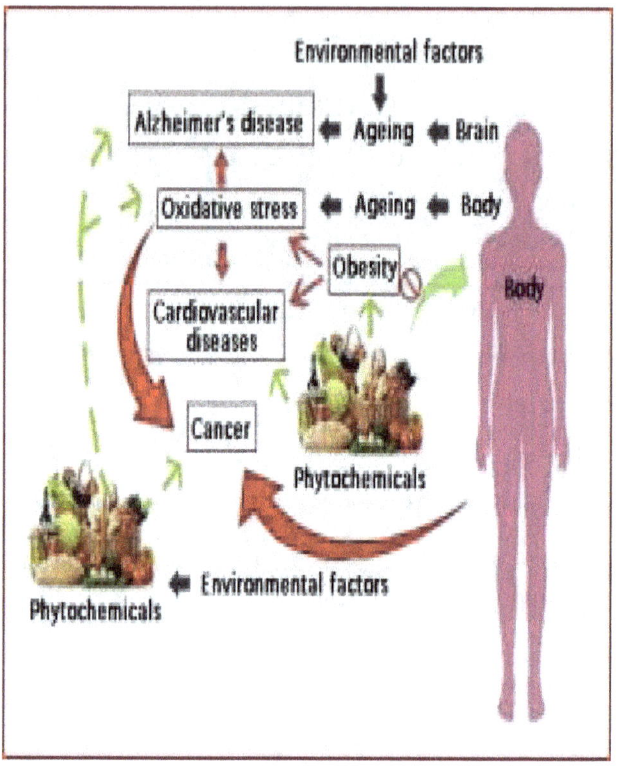

Vegetarianism is advocated for the traditional yogi and spiritual seeker as a means of reducing cruelty to animals and other forms of life. Although a vegetarian diet is generally advised for the dedicated yogi, getting enough of the right nutrients while staying vegetarian can be tricky, so vegetarian yogis often need to develop some nutrition knowledge as well. If a student adopts a vegetarian diet without first learning about proper nutrition, they may develop a host of unwanted health issues that will detract from their yoga practice.

For instance, one needs to understand proteins and their constituent amino acids if they intend to go on a vegetarian diet. Proteins are the body's primary structural components, making them vital to both development and health. Proteins are also present in plant materials, although they are categorized as "incomplete" due to the fact that they lack a sufficient quantity of several essential amino acids. Therefore, in order to get the healthiest possible "complete" protein from a plant-based diet, it is necessary to combine two different sources of amino acids. Due to the high concentration of essential amino acids it contains, meat is considered "complete" and necessitates no additional supplementation.

Meat is a staple in the diets of the young and the growing, as well as the sick and the weak, according to Oriental medicine. The concept of moderation and common sense applies here as well; eating too much meat can be just as harmful as eating too little. Meat is considered an essential component for healthy blood and abundant Qi. It's not always the case that eating meat means you're contributing to the suffering of another creature. Meat eaters can easily purge the negative karmas associated with their meat consumption by practicing appreciation and eating with awareness. Only an extremely small percentage of the population, according to Oriental medicine, is able to thrive on a raw vegetarian diet. Such a person is characterized by their robust health, muscular physique, and ferocious appetite. Though for most of us, adopting only a raw and vegetarian diet without proper education in nutrition and a suitable body type can cause unnecessary disturbance and deficiency in our Qi and blood stores.

It is suggested that fasting be done once a year. Detoxifying the mind is more important than the body when it comes to fasting. Fasting helps people overcome their dependence on food and other pleasure-seeking behaviors. Therefore, the yogi who fasts works to develop a strong willpower, which has far-reaching positive effects.

The condition of your internal organs can be accurately assessed by monitoring the frequency and consistency of your bowel movements. It's vital to take a moment to describe the ideal bowel movement because the subject rarely comes up in conversation.

Having a bowel movement once a day is generally regarded a positive indicator, and having that bowel movement before breakfast is the recommended time. The perfect poop is a shade of brown, neither too dry (as in pebble-like) nor too wet and loose. A bowel movement ought to be speedy, effortless, and require minimal wiping afterward. There shouldn't be any odor that causes the paint to chip either. Seeking professional medical aid to get your digestive system back on track is a good idea if you notice indicators of irregular or unhealthful bowel movements on a regular basis. You can get some help from an acupuncturist, herbalist, naturopath, or conventional medical doctor. While it's understandable that you'd rather avoid discussing this with your doctor, you should know that ignoring it could lead to serious consequences.

Constipation is a common symptom of an unbalanced modern diet and lifestyle. More physical activity, cutting back on breads, pastas, and other heavy foods, and supplementing with digestive tonics and stimulants like chile, lemon water, or apple cider vinegar will typically alleviate the resulting energy stagnation.

The inability to "let go" emotionally might appear physically as constipation. More information on this topic can be found in the book's Metal Element chapter. It is recommended that you consult a medical professional if you are unable to alleviate your constipation with self-care measures.

Fundamentals of the Oriental Dietary Approach:

Keep your satiety at 70-80%. Overeating drains vitality and wreaks havoc on the digestive system and spleen. The cerebral exercise is beneficial as well. A lack of mental equilibrium and a fixation on the senses are also indicators of compulsive overeating.

Mindfully, slowly, with few interruptions, and with a focus on your chewing.

Keep food temperatures moderate. This includes things like ice water and ice cream, both of which should be avoided. Foods cooked over open flames, foods that have been dried out, and foods that have been highly spiced should also be avoided.

Well-cooked foods, such as soups, stews, congees, and casseroles, are suggested in most situations, and especially in the event of illness, weakness, old age, or impaired digestion. Raw food diets are only sustainable for long durations by persons with a particularly robust constitution.

The serious yogi is advised to adopt a vegetarian diet; nevertheless, they should also learn about proper nutrition in order to prevent energy and blood deficits.

Meat is generally advised, particularly for children and the sick and weak.

The state of your internal organs can be accurately determined by observing their output. Constipation, diarrhea, or persistently loose stools are all conditions that need medical attention. Dietary changes, the use of digestive tonics, and the incorporation of more physically active routines are all viable options. If none of these measures help, medical attention should be sought.

The Organ-Related Muscles

In the '60s and '70s, we learned thanks to the efforts of Dr. George Good heart, a chiropractor, that each meridian in Chinese medicine. The energy system is intimately connected to the body's musculature and nervous system. Therefore, if a meridian is 'out' or not flowing normally, the associated muscle will not be working as it should, resulting in diminished neuromuscular activity. Thus, it was discovered that restoring the meridian would restore full muscle function, and restoring muscle function would likewise restore the meridian. A new dimension has been introduced to the treatment of energy dysfunction and the understanding of disease in the body thanks to this remarkable finding.

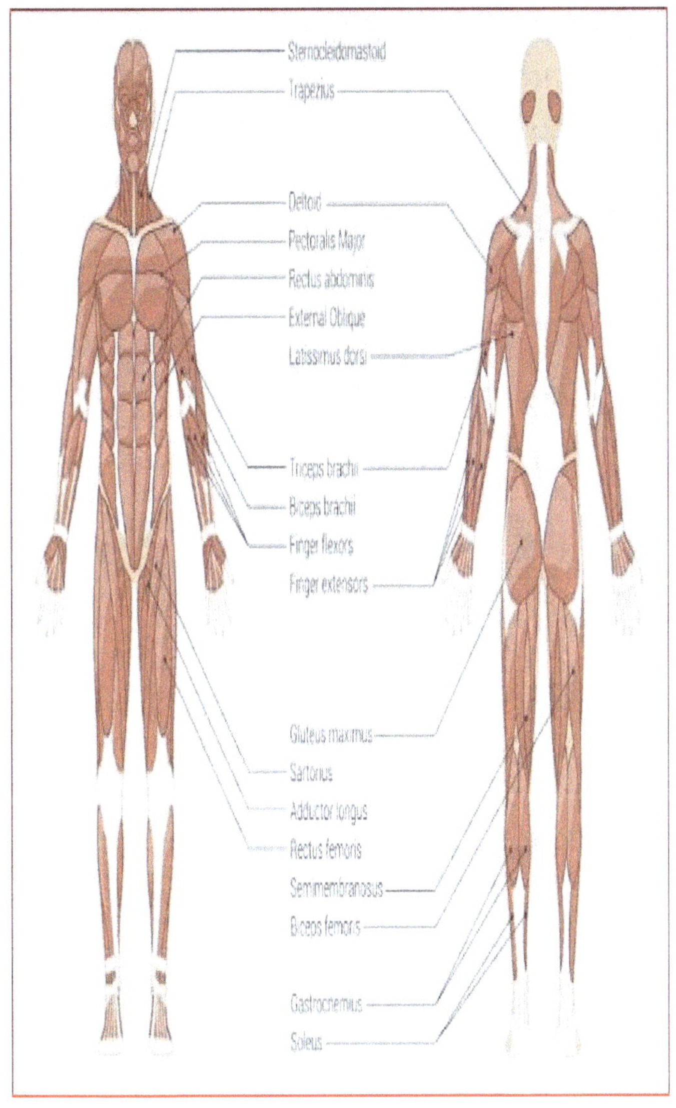

Asanas (postures) or any other form of movement training that targets certain areas of the body can be used to restore the proper energetic flow through our systems once we have learned the muscles connected with the meridians and the location of the meridians themselves. In subsequent chapters, the yoga asanas suggested for each meridian are discussed in detail.

The Basics of Oriental Yoga

Every yoga tradition places more weight on some aspects of the yogic lifestyle than others. This is not meant to be exclusive of other forms of yoga; rather, it is an attempt to highlight particular facets of yoga.

Change Always Prevails (Contemplations, Feelings, Events, Times of Year, etc.)

The yogi learns to detach from the material world because he or she realizes that change is the only constant. The yogi acknowledges form as it appears, but since he or she knows its actual essence, he or she lets it dissolve without holding on to it. The yogi must eventually ask themselves, "What is it that does not change?"

Embrace the Circulation of Life

We are privileged observers, privy to the unfolding of the universe's immensely well-planned process of consciousness evolution. We can only find peace and trust in the world as it is when we give up trying to manipulate or alter it to fit our ideals. When we have faith in this procedure, we are free to enjoy life and the here and now. To experience everything of life unfolding as it is, without having to put wrongness or rightness onto it, our perspective is likewise altered and the penetration of the smallness is transcended.

Happiness at Its Core (Under the Influence of Emotions)

Underneath the surface of our complex emotional lives lies an innate, default quality of existence: joy. It is fundamentally formless and yet possesses great subtlety and strength. Joy is revealed when the mind is purified and real sight is accomplished, penetrating all of the diverse forms and feelings.

Hara represents the human body, the heart represents the human emotional state, and the third eye represents the human spiritual state.

The Hara, or Dan Tien in Chinese, is the region directly below the belly button that is considered the physical center of the human body.

The third eye is the seat of the soul, whereas the heart is the nerve center for the mind and emotions. Within these three primary domains, the yogi cultivates presence, awareness, and space, with the Hara serving as the foundation that provides grounding for the other two domains.

Act as a Witness

The yogi is unaffected by his or her sensory impressions, including the mental activity that goes on around him or her, because he or she has adopted the perspective of an objective observer. As he or she becomes more proficient at this practice, the yogi will eventually be able to merge with the one who is witnessing all phenomena, having first investigated the one who is witnessing the senses.

Don't Hurt Anyone

Causing no damage not only helps maintain the vitality of all living things, but it also aids in the purging of negative karma and the strengthening of positive karma. In time, it becomes clear to the spiritual aspirant that nonviolence is a natural state of being, and so one makes the adjustment out of free will and compassion rather than out of obligation or fear.

The inclination to respond emotionally or physically to a situation as it develops is what creates karma. When these responses are reinforced, they give rise to more of the same, thereby perpetuating the cycle of karma. The yogi is free from the effects of karma when he or she has reached a state of non-reactivity and understanding regarding feelings and experiences.

Being able to take both good and bad feedback positively

Accepting, observing, and stopping to feed negativity is a yogic practice since it is a normal aspect of the human condition. This perspective shifts the stigma associated with unpleasant emotions and thoughts by redefining them as a source of energy that can be channeled toward personal development. Therefore, both positive and negative states can be used to purge old karma and advance one's own self-awareness.

Strength of Character and Will are Essential

The yogi knows that one's own thoughts and actions have the most significant influence in shaping one's experience of the world. It takes guts to look in the mirror and determination to keep your focus on mental hygiene and solidifying your place in the real world.

Constantly giving up and letting go

Only through living in the here and now can we experience true vitality. If we keep living in the past or anxiously anticipating an unknown future, we will never be fully present in the here and now. Surrendering what comes without adding further commentary is the key to staying present in the moment. By doing so, we can let go of whatever emotions, ideas, or bodily sensations may be present at any one time and instead focus on what is happening right now.

To Love and Be Loved, Existence Is All That's Required

To love someone or something unconditionally, one must let go of the urge to have a justification for doing so. When one realizes that simply being is enough, loving others and oneself becomes a natural response to God's gift of life.

Guidelines for a Yoga Lesson

It is important to discuss the major features included in an Oriental yoga style class that a student may attend because yoga is typically first encountered in a yoga class setting. The information in this chapter can help students prepare for classroom situations and better understand the rationale for certain classroom routines. The book also intends to help yoga instructors and teachers learn how to lead a class in the traditional Oriental yoga tradition.

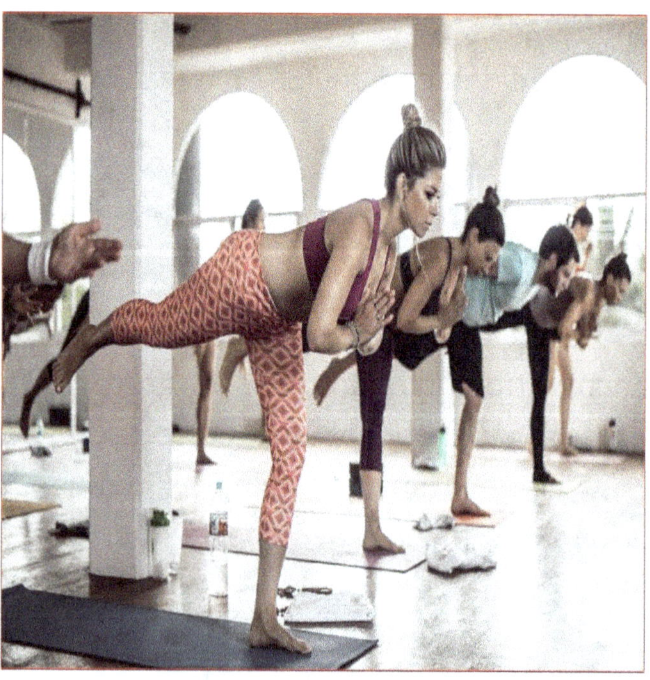

Loosen up

The importance of getting the body ready for practice cannot be overstated. Due to the widespread belief that modern man has no spare time, warming up is often neglected. The mind, the breath, and the flow of Qi and blood throughout the body can all benefit greatly from a good warm-up. One of the key goals of warming up is to induce a state of tranquility, as this allows the body and nervous system to relax and the body's energies to flow more freely, so enhancing subsequent practice. Mild warm-ups should ideally last between 20 and 30 minutes.

Mutual letting go

There are around 300 joints in the human body, with only seven being considered critical. These are the seven main joints:

-One's Ankles

- Knees

- Hips

-Head and Shoulders

- Bend your elbows

-and the wrists

- Neck

When two bones meet, that's called a joint. Joints are supported and able to move in a wide range of motion thanks to shock-absorbing cartilage, connective tissue, fibrous tissue, and fluids that keep bones at a safe distance from one another. A nutritious diet and most yoga practices can help by maintaining the health and hydration of this cartilage and fibrous tissue. Stagnation of Qi and blood is common in the joints, which are considered sacred sites in Chinese medicine. Stagnation of Qi and blood in the joints causes pain and muscle weakness, both of which increase the risk of injury. Therefore, it is crucial to include some joint release exercises in your warm up routine, targeting at least a few of the primary joints. Here are some tips for loosening up those joints.

Ankles

First, while lying on your back, begin slowly rotating your ankles in a circle.

Second, merely use 60-70 percent of your potential instead of the full 100.

Third, practice making fluid motions rather than sweeping ones.

Fourth, after one minute, begin to reverse direction.

Fifth, allow yourself to relax and shake it off.

Knees

1. Stand with your feet together and your knees bent. Kneel down with your hands on your knees and begin to make circular motions with your legs. Once more, you've only used 60–70% of your potential.
2. After one minute, switch the circles' polarity.

3. After two minutes, get up and give yourself a good shake to relieve tension.

Hips

1. Put your hands on your hips while you're standing. The distance between your feet should be equal to the breadth of your hips.

2. Begin making little, circular motions with your hips. Once more, don't go beyond 60-70 percent of your limit. Try to have the arcs as even as possible.

3. Turn around after one minute and go the other way.

4. When you're done, take a step back into a neutral stance and drop your arms.

Shoulders

1. Stand with feet hip-width apart and slowly move your shoulders forward,

up, back, and down. Don't go over 70% of your limit.

2. Do the move at least ten times, focusing on making it more and more fluid each time. Sharp pains will cause you to react violently, so use much smaller circles.

3. Change directions and go counterclockwise after 5-10 laps.

4. Relax your shoulder and give yourself a good shake when you're done.

Hands and Elbows

This is related to the last topic because when you move your wrist, you also move your elbow.

1. While standing, interlace your fingers and make a gentle, circular motion with your hands. Again, don't go over 70% of your limit.

2. After one minute, switch directions.

3. The fingers interlaced, but the elbows out to the side, as if resting the hands and forearms on a chest-height desk.

4. Then, using your arms and wrists, make a wavelike motion (this is the 1980s wave dance). Keep going like this for a minute.

5. After a minute, give waving the other way a shot.

6. After one minute, let your arms hang loosely at your sides.

Neck

You shouldn't use your full range of motion while doing these neck joint releases. Keep your effort level between 60 and 70 percent of maximum.

1. While standing, begin making small circles with your neck by gently bringing your chin forward, then to one side, up towards the sky a little bit, then back to the other side. Carry on making these soft neck circles for a while. Again, it's more important to pay attention to

the fluidity of the motion than the magnitude of it.

2.   After one minute, you should make a U-turn.

3. After one minute in each direction, you can unwind and take it easy.

1. You can do something very close to the standing position while lying on your back. Move your chin in soft, round motions. Move your chin in toward your chest, to one side, up toward the ceiling, and then to the opposite side.

2. Keep going in a circle for a minute before switching directions.

3.   When you're finished, let your head settle into its new position with ease and release.

Pranayama

Pranayama is the practice of directing one's breath to effect a shift in one's Qi. Although there are hundreds of different pranayama techniques in yoga, the practice of any one of them is not given much weight in traditional Eastern yoga. The focus is not on forcing or controlling the breath, but on cultivating a more efficient and aware breathing pattern that arises on its own as a result of regular asana, relaxation, and meditation.

Humans should try to breathe via their noses as much as possible. When at rest and not using the mouth for any purpose, supporting nasal breathing by placing the tip of the tongue on the roof of the mouth can help. A relaxed jaw and better skull-on-spine equilibrium are two additional benefits of this tongue posture. Nasal breathing offers many advantages over mouth breathing. Those things are:

1. By the time the air reaches the lungs, it has been adequately warmed and filtered.
2. Helps you breathe more slowly and relax your muscles and mind.

3. Aids in maintaining a healthy blood ph level.

4. Improves sleep quality by decreasing episodes of snoring and apnea.

5. Keeps the nerves in the nose alive and engaged, which improves our sense of smell.

6. The increased resistance to air pressure improves the flexibility and strength of the lung tissues.

7. Facilitates the storing and dispersal of kinetic energy.

8. Maintains mental acuity and performance.

It relieves stress on the facial and neck muscles and aids in keeping the head in proper alignment with the spine.

The average modern person has a habit of breathing too heavily. This person takes too many breaths in and doesn't release enough of them. This causes systemic physiologic disruption, which in turn sets off an inflammatory response and gives rise to respiratory issues like asthma. Therefore, ailments like asthma are amenable to treatment and even cure via methods like yoga.

Poor breathing techniques are also a major cause of anxiety-related illnesses. The mind's energy can be easily managed and repressed by the practice of effective breathing, which entails taking deeper, slower breaths.

When practicing relaxation and meditation, it's helpful to recognize that the breath's rhythm will change on its own over time, and to let it reorganize itself without forcing anything.

When practiced from a young age, efficient and appropriate breathing can strengthen the muscles linked with the mechanics of breathing, improve overall vitality, and pave the way for a more active and energized adult self. Activities like swimming and learning to play wind instruments can help children develop efficient and appropriate breathing at an early age.

Sound

Because of their profound effects on deepening the breath, soothing the mind, and releasing emotional and psychological pressures and other natural human noises during the yoga practice are always encouraged and advocated in Oriental yoga.

Mantras are effective tools for calming the mind and body by encouraging a slower, deeper breath and easing stress. The consequences of concentrating on and practicing any given mantra are identical, thus it really doesn't matter which one is chosen. On the other hand, the following mantras have proven to be really helpful to me personally.

Song: "On Mani Padme Hum"

Said in a chant: "Nam Myoho Renge Kyo"

Sutra of the Heart

Saa Hum

Chi Kung (Qi Gong)

Qi Gong, often known as "energy work," is the ancient Chinese practice of balancing and energizing one's internal and external Qi energy. When combined with yoga asana, Qi Gong offers a subtle yet potent energetic practice. Qi Gong, which has been described as a yin practice, and yoga asana, which has been described as a yang practice, are complementary to one another.

Some of Qi Gong's most notable advantages are:

1. Soft on the limbs
2. Feeds and lubricates the joints
3. Promotes healthy and balanced circulation of energy
4. Encourages healthy breathing

5. Increases receptivity to the bodily experience of Qi

6. The effect on the nerve system is very soothing.

7. Helps rewire the brain and reorganize muscular movement patterns for dramatically improved performance.

Because Qi Gong involves learning an entirely new way to move one's body, it takes time and effort to master the movements involved in it. This means that it typically takes a few months of consistent classroom practice for most students to begin "getting it" or "feeling it." Therefore, it is reasonable to assume that the amount we can learn about Qi Gong forms from a book like this is restricted. Practicing Qi Gong. However, I think it's important to discuss Qi Gong's fundamentals because of its central role in Oriental Yoga and in general energy cultivation.

Some of Qi Gong's guiding ideas are:

1. Always keep the joints supple and gently rounded (never lock out the joints) to facilitate the free flow of Qi.

2. Only use 60–90% of your maximum effort. Do not overwork yourself, as this can deplete your Qi.
3. Breathing and bodily movement should be in perfect time with one another.
4. Focus on the motion itself rather than the destination.
5. It's a constant motion that keeps going till told to stop.
6. Flow like water; nature and animal imagery is encouraged.
7. Relax; mother nature never hurries
8. At some point, you won't even have to think about making those motions; they'll just happen.

Any time you feel tired or anxious is a good time to practice Qi Gong, whether it be at the start of a class, right when you wake up, at the end of a class, or any other time.

If you want to study the fundamentals of Qi Gong, a video will serve you far better than this book. As a result, checking out YouTube is something you should do right now. Try Googling "Qi Gong for Beginners" to find a variety of free videos that will teach you the fundamentals of Qi Gong and get you started practicing right away. If you want personalized guidance from a skilled teacher, signing up for a series of local Qi Gong or Tai Chi courses is your best bet.

Asana

There are many benefits to performing yoga asanas (postures). In Oriental yoga, increasing one's physical flexibility is not the ultimate goal and is not indicative of a high level of practice. More crucial than physical flexibility is the ability to stay equanimous (steady, balanced, unmoved) in the face of pleasant and unpleasant sensations, both of which can be induced by yoga asanas.

The following are some of the functions of asanas:

1. The strengthening and regulation of the practitioner's Qi, blood, and vital energy

2. To prevent disease and pain by maintaining a fit and well-aligned body.

3. Reduce external disturbances during meditating.

4. To liberate pent-up emotions and sensations from the body's cellular memory

5. To develop one's own concentration, resolve, and resolve

Thinking and Reflection

To meditate in the classical sense, one must take a seated position and practice concentration techniques. The ability to focus on one task at a time is greatly improved via regular meditation practice. Concentration lays the groundwork for additional mental-based training by making it much easier for the mind to penetrate any task it is assigned.

A state of mind that is rooted in the present moment is what is meant by "meditation" in its colloquial definition. The nervous system can be trained to become more accustomed to the meditative state by beginning with the more formal practices of meditation. With practice, we can go about our days in a state of meditation and present-moment awareness, and eventually, this way of being will become second nature.

Contemplation is distinct from meditation in that it involves the examination of authoritative sources, such as the writings of saints or the words of the Bible. The practitioner then merely meditates on a single word, phrase, or line from a holy scripture. A re-contextualization of the phrase or line of sacred text in the practitioner's mind is intended to lead to the eventual realization of its entire reality. To contemplate is not to overthink or analyze; rather, it is to keep something in one's thoughts and give it time to "cook." Effective contemplation requires time and isolation, allowing the mind to zero in on a single subject for as long as it takes. More formal meditational practice may be appropriate until a higher capacity for concentration has been acquired if the mind is full and mental resources are distributed during contemplation.

CHAPTER 4

GROUNDWORK IN PHILOSOPHY

Yoga is not only a set of practices, but also a body of thought and belief. Our experience of the universe and ourselves, as well as our connections to all other things, can be better understood via the study and practice of yoga. Each theoretical tradition has its own take on how the world came to be and what our place in it should be, so there is a wide range of ways in which such connections and experiences can be interpreted.

IT'S NOT A RELIGION, YOGA

Although yoga has deep roots in Hindu culture, it is not the same thing as Hinduism, and you are not required to be Hindu to practice it. Each of the philosophical systems that make up yoga, with their own code of ethics, scriptures, physical postures, cleansing practices, breathing and meditation techniques, and so on, prescribes a unique way of life and relating to the world at large.

Select Your Preferred Yoga Style

Classical yoga, Advaita Vedanta, and tantra are the three primary worldviews that have emerged to form the basis of Hatha yoga in the West today. Almost every current yoga system can be traced back to one of these Indian schools of thought, providing a foundation for the practice and the wide variety of classes offered. Everything about a class—from the instructor's demeanor to the emphasis placed on different aspects of character—is shaped by the worldview to which the style adheres. Understanding the following three philosophical views will help you choose a yoga style that serves your purpose, even if the presence of a spiritual philosophy isn't always obvious in class.

Patanjali's Yoga or Classical Yoga

The Yoga Sutras, written over 2,000 years ago by the Indian philosopher Patanjali, are the foundation for the vast majority of yoga practices in the West. This practice is known as Ashtanga yoga (ashta meaning "eight" and anga meaning "limb"). The scholar gathered and organized the most crucial concepts, philosophies, and practices of the yoga tradition into 196 pithy aphorisms called sutras. Patanjali gave yoga its classical style by giving a formalized theoretical framework; the system of thought outlined in the Yoga Sutras is hence usually referred to as classical yoga.

Classical yoga is a dualistic philosophy because it separates spirit (purusha) and nature (prakriti), which are both real but never coexist. Your physical being, mental processes, and emotional experiences are all a part of nature's manifest, material plane. Spirit, on the other hand, is your genuine or highest Self and is limitless, absolute, and immutable. According to Patanjali, the source of all human distress is the mistaken belief that the self (including the physical body, the mind, and the emotions) are absolute. This link leads to narrow conceptions of the world and of who we are. One must rise above the material world in order to gain freedom from their restricted life and the misery that comes with it. Since your spirit (or true Self) is infinite and exists outside of time and space, nature is viewed as something to be overcome. To separate purusha from the diverse components of the physical world and for pure awareness to emerge naturally, one must have perfect mastery and control over one's body, mind, and emotions.

Ashtanga yoga has arrived. Patanjali's eightfold route to enlightenment begins with a moral compass and culminates in a state of spiritual transcendence by outlining a series of practices designed to help you detach your sense of yourself from your material existence. The path is depicted as an ascending ladder with eight progressively more difficult rungs, with the first two rungs (asanas and pranayama) serving as preparation for the more advanced rungs (concentration and meditation). To achieve complete mastery of one's ideas and emotions, one must first gain control over one's physical body and breathing, and then one's senses and mental fluctuations. The final step of Ashtanga yoga prepares the seeker for the ecstatic condition of pure existence, which occurs when the seeker spontaneously transcends prakriti and is absorbed into purusha.

Ashtanga Yoga

1. Yama (moral discipline) refers to a set of guiding principles for how we should act in various social contexts.
2. Niyama (self-restraint) refers to a set of specific rules of conduct about one's own physical and mental discipline that serve as guidelines for one's interactions with oneself.
3. Asana (yoga postures) are physical exercises that help you become more flexible and strong, and that also help you develop the self-control and concentration skills you'll need to meditate effectively.
4. Pranayama (breath control) refers to a set of techniques used to regulate one's breathing in order to gain control over prana, or vital life force.
5. The act of withdrawing one's senses from the exterior world in order to concentrate on one's own inner experience is known as pratyahara.
6. Dharana (concentration) is the single-minded attention attained after asana (postures), pranayama (breathing exercises), and pratyahara (withdrawal of the senses) have been practiced.
7. Dhyana (meditation) means "uninterrupted concentration" or "concentration without an object."

8. Samadhi, often known as ecstasy, is the highest level of contemplative absorption.

Meditation is at the heart of Patanjali's yoga, which is why it is frequently called the royal path or king (raja) yoga (Yoga Sutra 1.2: yoga chitta vritti nirodha [yoga is for the cessation of the mind's fluctuations]). Asana practice in yoga is only one of eight limbs that lead to enlightenment. Asana was historically meant to prepare the body for lengthy periods of seated meditation, but its ultimate purpose is to transcend the physical experience (the body is a tool used to realize that you are not your body at all but rather something absolute beyond relative form). The word "asana" from Sanskrit for "seat." Yoga asana practice is unnecessary after a learner has reached a more advanced level of practice and gained mastery over their physical body. Most contemporary yoga practices aim to integrate the eight limbs of Ashtanga into a single practice, which includes executing asana with self-discipline, breath control, and undivided focus. However, some systems continue to view asana as a technique and place more emphasis on seated meditation.

Advaita Vedanta

Swami Vivekananda, who lectured at the 1893 World's Fair in Chicago, exposed the Western world to Advaita Vedanta, one of the most prominent and influential sub schools of the Vedanta Indian school of thought. There are several well-known Hatha yoga traditions that trace their roots back to the Vedanta school of Indian philosophy, and there are also a growing number of Advaita Vedanta organizations and ashrams across the United States.

Philosophy in the Vedanta Tradition

Vedanta, which literally translates to "end of the Vedas," is the umbrella term for a variety of philosophical traditions that draw their worldview from the Upanishads.

Advaita (nondual) Vedanta is a monist philosophy which, in contrast to traditional yoga, asserts that there is only one actual reality, Brahman, which is absolute, omnipresent, transcendent, and eternal. Everything that changes over time, such as differences we perceive (duality), is a fabrication. Ignorance is thought to be at the basis of the illusion of the world and all its variety. Only One Exists. And your true nature is Brahman, the One.

Picture yourself on a dark road, about to pass a snake when it appears out of nowhere. You freeze up from fear of snakes, unable to move another muscle. The clouds part and the moon shines through, revealing the snake to be a rope rather than a dangerous foe. It is common in Advaita Vedanta to use the analogy of a snake and a rope to describe the nature of the relationship between Brahman and the manifest world: Just as you confused the snake and the rope, the universe is a conflation with Brahman; and just as the moon's light spontaneously revealed the rope beneath the snake's skin, so does true knowledge spontaneously reveal the oneness of reality beneath the veil of ignorance.

Because of this flawed self-understanding, Advaita Vedanta holds, we are born into bondage (the cycle of rebirths). Ignorance of our true nature and the unity of reality is the root cause of our pain. Moksha, or freedom from rebirth, can be achieved by a shift in perspective and an acceptance of one's essential identity as Brahman. This entails the same premise as classical yoga: that the physical body, the mind, and the emotions are not the true you, that the true you is the transcendental Self, and that emotional sorrow is the result of identification with the manifest nature. Advaita Vedanta, on the other hand, teaches that Moksha can be attained immediately upon opening to the actual knowledge of oneness and realizing that all sensations of duality are really a psychological illusion.

Advaita Vedanta's primary route is Jnana yoga, often known as the yoga of knowledge or wisdom. Advaitins who are interested in understanding their true nature can benefit from practicing Bhakti, Raja, Karma, and Hatha yoga; yet, only Jnana, pure knowledge, can bring one directly to Moksha. Introspective study of the Upanishads is claimed to lead to a direct realization of Brahman.

Neither of these nor that

Neti (which literally means "not this, not this") is the most widely practiced Advaita Vedanta technique. Neti is a method of negating all that is not Brahman, and it can be recited or repeated while meditation.

Tantra

Neither denying nor affirming the two prior schools of thought, Indian philosophical thought underwent a radical shift after the establishment of classical yoga and Advaita Vedanta, recognizing the supreme oneness of the universe and accepting the existence of both realities (relative and absolute). (Tantra, derived from Sanskrit, means "weave" or "loom.") The tantra school of thought integrated and developed the previous two concepts.

Everything in the universe is seen as supreme consciousness, and yet all differences are real, from the perspective of tantric nondualism, in which there is no duality between spirit (purusha) and matter (prakriti). Rather than denying the reality of opposites,

Tantra views the material universe as a collection of Divine manifestations or utterances. Since everything in the universe, from the most banal things to the most sublime, is made up of pure consciousness, there is nothing to go beyond and no barriers to overcome.

Tossing a Coin

There is no gap between the realm of supreme consciousness and the world of duality; they are only two sides of the same coin. The coin has two sides: the many expressing themselves as one, and the one doing the same.

For Tantrikas (followers of tantra), the body is not a hindrance but a blessing, and rebirth is seen not as a punishment but as a second chance at life. Nothing exists outside of consciousness, thus every moment is a chance to learn more about yourself. Your physique is not a barrier to your potential. Instead, the sublime can be felt as an ecstatic dance within your physical being. Asana is also a part of tantra, but with a twist. Unlike in classical yoga, where asana practice is seen as a means to an end (a stepping stone to transcendence), in liberation yoga, asana practice is seen as a celebration of your inherent freedom in this physical body in the present moment.

Asana, the practice of yoga postures, is commonly thought to originate from Patanjali's classical yoga (asana is the third limb of Ashtanga yoga), but Hatha yoga didn't emerge until the tantra movement came together, and some would argue that all modern styles of yoga are based in tantra despite being ascribed to classical yoga philosophy.

CHAPTER 5

REASONS FOR FEELING DOWN

Ayurveda teaches that joy is innate to the human condition. Most of us agree with you when we're alone with our thoughts. We have a deep-seated knowledge that our potential for happiness exceeds our actual experiences. We know there's a wellspring of joy and vigor within, but it's a resource we're having a hard time tapping into. We spend our lives aimlessly searching for the key that will open that safe, but we rarely find it.

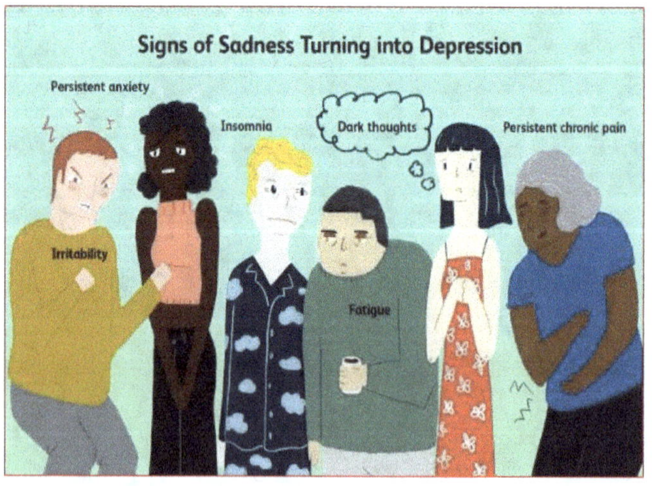

When did our joy disappear? The key to our inheritance is still in our possession; we simply cannot find it. We have forgotten that our pleasure is shaped by the cumulative effect of our decisions at every stage of life.

The sunflower must face the sun in order to survive. This ensures its continued existence and growth. We, on the other hand, have the capacity to reason, which provides us with alternatives. We forget, unlike the sunflower, that we are a part of nature and thus subject to its rules. Every day, we make poor decisions regarding our diet, amount of sleep, level of physical activity, and how we spend our time. It's not uncommon for people to make mistakes without intending to, but the physical consequences still stick. By doing so, we shut down our capacity for joy and foster the development of clinical depression. The silver lining is that our creations are reversible. We'll find the key, open the vault, and claim our rightful inheritance once we come to terms with the interconnectedness of our physical, mental, and spiritual selves.

Ayurveda Unconventional Methodology

Ayurveda provides benefits that conventional medicine and therapy are unable to treat. It explains how we bring about depression and how we might overcome it. Ayurveda toolkit is stocked with numerous effective methods for revitalizing our health and well-being. It can aid people at any point along the depressive spectrum. Ayurvedic remedies are tailored to the individual, so whether you have the blues, have suffered from depression, or just want to stay emotionally healthy, you can find something that works for you.

When compared to conventional medical theory, the Ayurvedic view of physiology has more in common with that of modern physicists. Human physiology is seen as a pattern of vibrations in a sea of consciousness (intelligence) by both ancient Vedic sages and modern quantum mechanics physicists. Sages and physicists, separated by thousands of years yet using similar language to explain the human condition in the cosmos.

When we view the human body through the lens of Ayurveda, our perspective shifts. To begin, we are cautioned by the Vedic sages against viewing ourselves as static entities. They say that all of reality is in a state of flux, a vast ocean of awareness. Second, they teach us that our bodies are only an extension of their surroundings. Everything in this ocean of consciousness influences and is influenced by us. Finally, ancients say that our bodies are nothing more than a vibrational pattern directed by an innate intellect.

Knowing how the natural world functions is crucial to grasping human physiology. Nature organizes everything. It is constructed in layers, and what we see with our eyes is only the manifest layer. There is a rational, orderly unfolding of the different strata of nature. Differently structured forms of energy become apparent when we peel back the layers of nature, from the visible to the invisible. To put it another way, energy is what drives our body.

However, this does not discount the fact that, at the manifest level, we are indeed corporeal beings. (You give off a substantial impression; you feel solid; you are solid.) But at a deeper level, you are one continuous energetic system, and every part of you has an effect on the whole. In order to properly promote health and wellness, it is necessary to learn how to treat the underlying layers of our physiology.

How Does Mood Disorder Develop?

Yes, depression is real. It might creep up on a person slowly, like water dripping into a basement, or it can slam into them quickly, like a raging windstorm. Genes, environment, and health all have a role in the development of depression. The toll that daily life takes on our bodies, minds, and spirits should not be minimized. No matter the cause, Ayurveda offers us hope by providing tools for warding off depression.

The Vedic sages aren't interested in discussing your cerebral cortex (or your mom, for that matter). The circulation of vital energy throughout your body is of paramount importance in their view. Physiological issues, such as depression, can arise when the flow of life-energy is restricted or hindered. This is due to the fact that energy is necessary for every action. Simply put, we are energy beings.

Illness occurs when the free flow of energy in our bodies is disrupted. This is the form that illness will take if we are susceptible to depression. The energy of life is what drives our thoughts and gives us the capacity to make things and feel good. A healthy mind is the driving force behind a healthy body. The transfer of life-energy from the environment into our bodies is reflected in how we feel emotionally, mentally, and physically.

Anything that prevents us from utilizing our available life-energy or drains it is a depressant. There are several causes, but ongoing stress is most prominent. The second is physiological aging, which may or may not coincide with chronological aging. It gets harder to protect against the damaging effects of stress as we get older, and we grow more prone to clogging up the channels in our energy system. Without regular and effective attention, this accumulation will weigh down our spirit.

Life-energy blockage can be understood through the application of a simple principle: as energy transformers, we take in information about the world through our five senses. In truth, we process all information that enters our brains through our senses. You are what you consume, quite literally. First, though, let's agree that "eat" means to take in and process whatever comes into one's physical, mental, and spiritual bodies.

Undigested material can cause disruption in any part of our being if our physical, mental, or emotional digestive function is subpar. We feel depressed because of the oppression we're experiencing.

Another key belief in Ayurveda is that human people, like all other forms of life and inorganic matter, should be treated as sacred. Our biological systems have biorhythms that are precisely timed to the cycles of the natural world. Despite our evolutionary progress, we still must obey the laws of nature.

But unlike other animals in nature, humans can consciously and subconsciously engage in behaviors that lead to physiological imbalances. It's not like any wild animals work 18-hour days or snack on pizza at 3 in the morning. In the long run, depression and other illnesses might result from repeated actions that go against nature's laws.

Deficiency of vital energy, accumulation of muck in our seamless energetic system, which blocks access to the free fl ow of our life - energy, and physiologic abnormalities are all contributors to depression.

How Can I Reverse My Mood Disorder?

Vitality, the antithesis of despair, must be manufactured. When your body is strong and full of life, you'll naturally feel happy. The inherent intelligence of the cosmos is the ultimate wellspring of energy. By highlighting the independent side of natural intellect, we generate life.

Unfortunately, as we age, we often become more set in our ways and fail to develop into the best versions of ourselves. Without outside help, people will naturally fall back on tried-and-true methods and routines. We wear grooves into the neural system through the repetition of thought, feeling, and action routines. Neurochemicals are released in response to mental and emotional processes and serve to organize our bodies. Because of the established framework, we are compelled to repeat actions. Because of this, some researchers have proposed that we develop a "addiction" to the ways in which we regularly think, feel, and act.

Changing our brain and metabolic pathways can help us overcome depression and bring about lasting happiness. This change in our psychological and physiological makeup allows us to express a wider range of feelings, thoughts, and actions. This growth motivates us in every way to be healthy and flourishing. According to Ayurveda, changing our mental and physiological habits requires more than just talking about it or thinking about it.

Ayurveda uses methods that revitalize the whole person, including the mind, body, and soul, to combat depression. These methods release stagnation, restore harmony, and energize the body. They are straightforward and simple to implement, making them highly practical.

There are some essential components shared by Ayurvedic approaches that serve as vitality agents. The first benefit is that they help us fall in step with the natural world. Second, if energy blocks are present, they trigger the body's purification mechanisms, assisting the individual in achieving mental and physical clarity. They also aid with digestion, allowing us to more effectively convert mental and emotional states as well as food into useful energy.

These treatments address the underlying causes of depression by operating at the level of awareness, the core of our being.

The following set of depression-fighting methods is meant to free our inherent healing capacity by making way for natural recovery:

1. Realize that the fundamental nature of your body, mind, and soul is consciousness. We talk about how everything in the cosmos may be traced back to awareness, the intellect that directs nature. We describe how the human

body is more than just a mass of stuff; it is also a vibratory pattern that arises from a field of energy. This idea has the potential to spark a paradigm shift that will completely alter the way depression is now treated medically.

2. Figure out how your depression manifests itself in your case. Taking an Ayurvedic view of depression allows for more nuanced evaluation of signs and symptoms. Inconsistencies in the body's fundamental elements are linked to certain ailments. There are three distinct varieties of depression—"airy," "burning," and "earthy"—each corresponding to a different kind of physiological imbalance.

We use a patient with Airy Depression, characterized by worry, as an example. In this case study, we examine Burning Depression, a form of the mood disorder marked by a constant outpouring of negative emotions. We also detail a case of Earthy Depression, characterized by emotional and physical apathy.

3. Improve your physical, mental, and spiritual absorption of food and experience. We demonstrate how depression affects not just the brain but the entire body and mind as well as

the spirit. Inadequate digestion of either food or life experiences might lead to depression. Either way, we can stifle joy and prevent energy from flowing freely. In order for our minds and bodies to work together efficiently, we need our digestive fire to be at full strength on every level.

4. Strengthen your body by sleeping well. Sleep and rest are crucial for overcoming depression. We talk about the restorative effects of meditation on the body and the nervous system on a daily basis.

We give examples of the negative effects of sleep deprivation on both the intellect and the body. Because of this strain, our energetic pathways become blocked or our bodies become out of whack. Moodiness is triggered by fatigue, and only extended sleep may lift it.

5. Try yoga positions and deep breathing exercises designed specifically for you. We can't expect a cookie-cutter approach to work for everyone suffering from depression. In this article, we explain how to overcome depression with deep breathing, physical activity, and yoga positions. We help you create a plan that is

tailored to how you experience depression. Breathing exercises, physical activity, and various yoga postures all have a stimulating effect on the body and mind. They help us both create and freely distribute our life force. Different strokes for different folks is the overarching theme of these sections. Choose the healing methods that work best for you.

6. Medicate with food. Food, according to Ayurveda, should be seen as "information packets" that bring us in touch with nature's innate wisdom. We talk about how the morsel at the end of our fork might hold the key to overcoming sadness. Just as important, we think, is the idea that it's not so much what we eat as it is how we eat that affects our physical, mental, and spiritual well-being.

7. Treat yourself with some meditation. In chapter 9, we emphasize the stress-relieving, energy-boosting, and awareness-widening benefits of regular meditation practice. We refer to scientific studies that have been repeated and found to be accurate in their conclusions about the efficacy of meditation as a treatment for depression.

Although there are many methods to increase energy, meditation is one of the most effective. Our natural ability to heal ourselves is activated by the practice of meditation. The deep sleep that results from this is essential for the body's own healing processes. It cleanses the whole person in a way that is both profound and delicate. It revs up our metabolic furnace, helping us digest food more efficiently. Most importantly, it gives us what is rightfully ours: a chance at joy and health.

Awakening the Healer within You

Try to remember the last time you got an infection, such a cold or stomach virus, and how miserable you felt. When did you first realize you were sick? Were there any early warning signs? If so, how did you deal with it? How did you find the most success? Can you draw any conclusions about your body's recuperative capacities from this experience? Do you know about the healing intelligence that guides wound healing in the body? If you want to start being your own doctor, where do you want to start?

CHAPTER 6

SO, WHY DAHN YOGA?

Stand up straight and take your place in the world. Those who don't feel any shame in themselves stand tall and keep their cool under pressure.

(From the ancient Korean religious literature) The Cham-jun-kye-kyung.

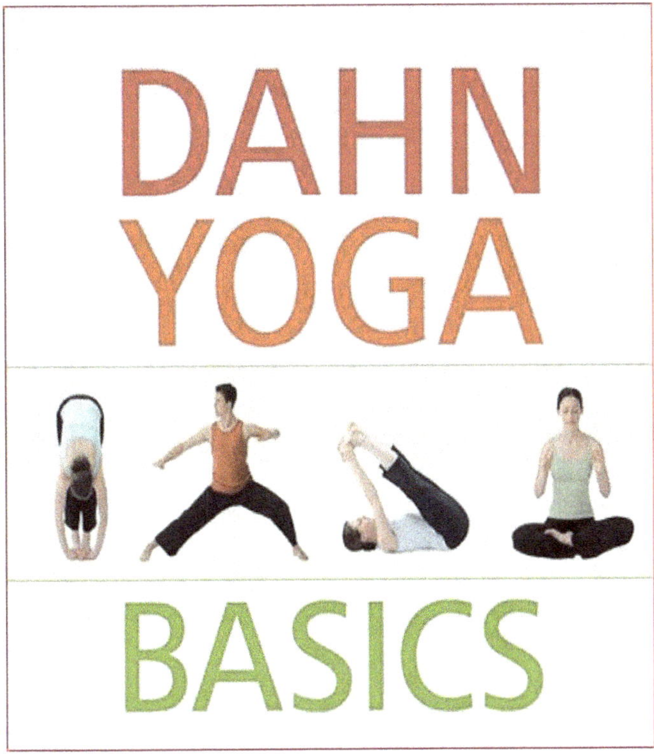

Dahn Yoga: What Is It?

Dahn Yoga is an all-encompassing practice that includes deep stretching, mindful breathing, and energy awareness instruction. The goal of this approach is to aid its practitioners in reaching their fullest potential.

Traditional practitioners of Dahn Yoga refer to it as "Dahnhak," which translates to "the study of energy." The Korean words "Dahn" and "Hak" mean "primal vital energy" (central to all forms of life) and "study of a particular theory or philosophy," respectively. Dahnhak practitioners are those who study the energy system to better themselves.

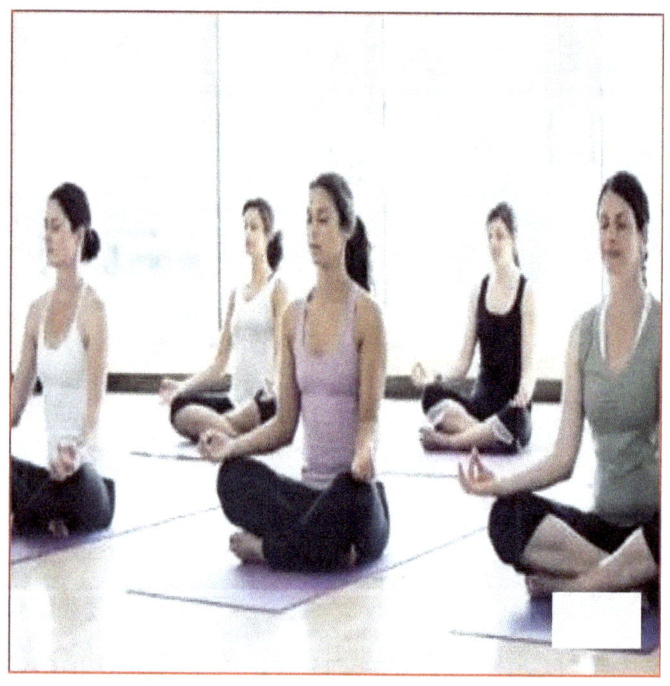

Dahn Yoga teaches students to read their own energy fields and use that as a means of self-expression. When the flow of energy within the body is encouraged, the body's own natural healing abilities are released. Practitioners can guide themselves back to peak health with regular practice. Using Ki, they are able to reclaim control of their bodies and minds.

However, the advantages of Dahn Yoga go far beyond mere physical fitness. To begin, Dahn Yoga's definition of "health" is extremely broad. A healthy individual doesn't just focus on physical fitness, but also on finding internal peace and contentment. Many devotees of Dahn Yoga claim to have experienced positive changes in their personal and professional lives, as well as the release of long-repressed emotions.

When a practitioner achieves his or her goal of a healthy life, he or she may decide to broaden his or her focus to include establishing mutually beneficial bonds with other people and with the natural world. This makes them better people overall and contributes to a more positive, peaceful environment.

In What Ways Does This Help?

Dahn Yoga was designed for people who desire to improve their life by increasing their mobility and achieving mental and physical equilibrium despite their demanding schedules. Dahn Yoga's simplicity and accessibility make it ideal for beginners, while its depth and complexity make it a worthy challenge for seasoned yogis. Dahn Yoga is open to everyone, regardless of gender, age, or physical ability. The following advantages are possible through consistent practice:

MIND AND BODY: The deep stretching and breathing exercises engage every muscle and joint in your body evenly to:

1. Improve your range of motion and equilibrium.
2. Enhance your oxygen intake, stamina, and overall health.
3. Increase your muscle strength and bone density.
4. Assist in keeping your metabolism in check.
5. Strengthen heart and blood vessel health.
6. Facilitate bodily pain management.
7. Improve blood flow to all of the body's systems.

IN YOUR HEAD: Dahn Yoga aims to integrate body posture, breath, and consciousness. This is the main distinction between Dahn Yoga and other types of stretching. Focusing on your posture, slowing your breathing, and being fully present in the moment might help you:

1. Help you unwind and remain composed in high-pressure circumstances.
2. Help you learn to concentrate without distractions.
3. Promote optimistic thinking and self-love.
4. Bring about a sense of calm and equilibrium.

FOR THE SOUL. Dahn Yoga can be practiced for no other reason than to improve one's health. This system, however, is all-encompassing, covering not only the cerebral and physiological, but also the spiritual dimensions of man. Meditation and spiritual awakening thanks to Dahn Yoga practice.

1. Tune into your senses and learn to tune in to your body, your emotions, and your environment.
2. Make you feel at one with the world and with nature.
3. Assist you in identifying and recovering your life's driving motivation.

What Makes Dahn Yoga Special?

While Dahn Yoga shares similarities with other mind-body practices, it is distinct in three ways:

1. **THE CONTROL AND APPLICATION OF POWER:** Dahn Yoga centers on the belief that one's energy is the link between their physical and mental selves. Through energy work, practitioners strengthen the link between their minds and bodies and gain a more in-depth understanding of their physical selves.

Dahn Yoga consists of the five phases of generating, storing, directing, and dissipating energy. Students begin by learning to sense and store energy in the body's key energy nodes. There is an increase in energy flow throughout the body as clogged energy channels gradually free up during the process of developing a sensation of energy. Once practitioners learn to harness and direct energy, they are able to heal their bodies naturally and gain mastery over their feelings, thoughts, and routines.

Dahn Yoga practice can be carried out despite a lack of vitality. However, when students feel energy, they encounter the true nature of Dahn Yoga, and the training itself becomes more joyful and grows into an experience with many dimensions.

2. BODY-MIND INTEGRATION IMPROVEMENT: According to Dahn Yoga, the brain is more than just an organ; it is the hub of the entire body's energy system. Dahn Yoga teaches its students to focus their attention and energy in order to improve their lives and the lives of those around them. But the brain's potential isn't just for bettering oneself in the abstract. The human mind is capable of both sowing discord and fostering intolerance, and nurturing harmony and well-being.

3.   HEALTH CARE THAT IS SELF-MANAGED AND HOLISTIC. In addition to physical health, the Dahn Yoga curriculum emphasizes the development of healthier emotional habits. In particular, it has a lot of features that help people communicate and engage better with others. It's also useful for breaking other bad routines like smoking and overeating. This is made feasible by the core tenets of Dahn Yoga and its methodical approaches to training, which will be discussed in further depth below.

How Did This Get Started?

Dahn Yoga has been practiced for thousands of years in Korea. It was originally conceived as a means of fostering the intellectual and physical growth of Korea's populace. It was done on a regular basis so that individuals might stay healthy and grow into more perfect versions of themselves. This style of teaching was used and passed down from generation to generation by wise individuals until around two thousand years ago. Dahnhak helped the Korean people over hundreds of years, improving their health and uniting them politically. Unfortunately, the Korean people did not succeed in maintaining the Dahnhak custom.

Ilchi Lee, on a quest for enlightenment and self-control, rediscovers and updates the ancient practice. While visiting a small park in Anyang, Korea, he met a stroke patient and began instructing them in Dahnhak. The pioneering Dahn center had its beginnings in Seoul, Korea in 1985. Since then, the program has gone global, with over 600 locations now delivering Dahn Yoga to a total of over 200,000 people. Thousands of public parks, schools, assisted living institutions, and university campuses in Korea, the United States, Canada, Japan, and other nations continue the tradition of providing the activities to their visitors.

How to Begin?

1. **LOCATION:** Dahn Yoga can be practiced anywhere; a special studio is not required. It's equally at home in either a gym or a park. The training techniques discussed here are suitable for use anywhere, from the office to a roadside rest area. You should practice Dahn Yoga in a regular location for the best results. Find a place with low background noise and enough room to spread out. Keep the temperature at a comfortable level, neither too hot nor too cold.

2. **CLOTHING:** Dress in a way that allows you to move freely and easily. To keep dry and comfortable, wear garments manufactured from a natural material. If you can, try to do your workouts barefoot.

3. **SCHOOLING PERIOD:** Two to three hours after a meal is the optimal time to hit the gym. Dahn training involves bending the body forward and backward as well as twisting it side to side, which may be uncomfortable if

you have recently eaten. A morning workout is a terrific way to jumpstart the day, but you should train whenever is most convenient for you.

If at all feasible, commit to a specific amount of training time, preferably between one and one and a half hours. However, if this is not possible, at least 20 minutes of training per day is recommended. If you can't work out every day, try to get in at least two or three sessions every week. The best method to learn Dahn Yoga is to acquire training and direction from a professional instructor at a Dahn center, however this book will serve as a basic introduction.

"THE END"

www.ingramcontent.com/pod-product-compliance
Lightning Source LLC
Chambersburg PA
CBHW051755250726
48659CB00001B/422